ADVANCED SKINCARE TREATMENTS FOR BEGINNERS

Professional Techniques, Anti-Aging Solutions, And Custom Routines For Radiant Body

DR SAWYER DIEGO

DISCLAMER

Nothing in this book should be interpreted as medical advice; it is meant exclusively for educational reasons. Regarding their specific health issues and treatment options, readers are urged to speak with licensed healthcare professionals. The publisher and author disclaim all liability for any errors or omissions in the material provided, as well as for any negative effects that may arise from using or abusing the information. Although every attempt has been taken to guarantee that the material in this book is correct as of the date of publishing, new research may have superseded some of the content because medical knowledge is always changing. It is recommended that readers confirm the most recent medical recommendations and guidelines. The reader of this book undertakes to release the author and publisher from any claims or liabilities resulting from the use of this information, and understands and accepts the inherent risks connected with healthcare decisions.

TABLE OF CONTENTS

ABOUT THE BOOK

For those who want to take their skincare regimens above and beyond the basics, "Advanced Skincare Treatments for Beginners" is an invaluable resource. This book addresses a wide range of skin diseases and concerns, giving readers thorough knowledge and useful insights into advanced skincare treatments.

The book's main focus is on the significance of comprehending basic skincare concepts, which provides a strong foundation for exploring more sophisticated procedures. By giving readers a comprehensive rundown of typical skincare issues, the author helps them better understand their personal skin needs and the advantages of getting professional advice.

Comprehensive coverage of efficient skincare techniques is ensured by the inclusion of in-depth insights into a variety of cutting-edge treatments, including chemical peels, microdermabrasion, microneedling, laser treatments, anti-aging protocols, and acne therapies. Every treatment is carefully examined, including its mechanisms and advantages as well as useful factors like safety measures, preparatory measures, and after-treatment care. This method gives readers the information they need to make wise decisions about their skincare journey in addition to educating them.

The book also emphasizes how important it is to have reasonable expectations and recognize the distinctions between basic and expert skincare techniques. It draws attention to the part skincare specialists play in customizing treatments to suit each patient's unique skin type and condition to maximize benefits and reduce dangers.

Concerns and commonly asked issues about skin sensitivity, cost of treatments, and DIY safety are addressed so that readers are equipped to make informed decisions about their skincare. The book's dedication to improving long-term skin health and vitality is highlighted by the emphasis on maintenance and long-term benefits.

"Advanced Skincare Treatments for Beginners" is more than simply a manual—it's a partner in helping you achieve beautiful, healthy skin through well-informed decisions and professional advice. It acts as a guide for anyone looking to improve their skincare regimens with treatments that have scientific backing and encourages a pro-active approach to skincare that puts efficacy, safety, and long-term skin wellbeing first.

CHAPTER ONE

ADVANCED SKINCARE TREATMENTS OVERVIEW

KNOWING THE FUNDAMENTALS OF SKINCARE

Understanding the foundational ideas of skincare is essential before pursuing more sophisticated skincare procedures. Modern methods and therapies are developed based on these fundamental ideas. Understanding your skin type is essential to basic skincare since it determines the products and routines that work best for you. For example, different care is needed for oily skin than for dry or sensitive skin types. Basic skin care practices like cleansing, moisturizing, and protecting against the sun help to maintain skin health and set the stage for more specialized treatments.

Furthermore, simplicity and consistency are emphasized by fundamental skincare concepts. The foundation of healthy skin care practices is creating a daily routine that involves moisturizing to nourish the skin, protecting it from UV damage with sunscreen, and gently washing to eliminate pollutants. Comprehending the functions of components like retinoids, hyaluronic acid, and antioxidants facilitates the selection of cosmetics that target particular issues like acne, pigmentation, or aging. Beginning with these foundational techniques, novices create a strong foundation for progressing to more specific treatments catered to their skincare objectives.

THE VALUE OF CUTTING-EDGE THERAPIES

Targeting certain difficulties with more involved techniques and ingredients, advanced skincare treatments offer customized remedies that go beyond conventional skincare routines. These procedures are intended to deal with troublesome conditions like wrinkles, fine lines, hyperpigmentation, and acne scars that might not be sufficiently resolved by over-the-counter remedies. The value of advanced therapies is found in their capacity to produce more pronounced and focused outcomes, frequently using operations like chemical peels, microdermabrasion, or laser therapy.

Furthermore, when administered by qualified personnel, cutting-edge treatments are safe and successful since they are supported by clinical efficacy and scientific studies. To stimulate collagen formation and encourage cellular renewal, they frequently contain larger concentrations of active substances or technology that permeate deeper layers of the skin. This cutting-edge method can greatly enhance skin tone, texture, and appearance overall, giving people a more radiant and youthful complexion.

AN OVERVIEW OF TYPICAL SKINCARE ISSUES

Before attempting advanced skincare treatments, it's critical to identify the main skincare issues that most people have. These worries range widely and include conditions like acne, which can affect adults and teenagers owing to heredity or hormonal changes. Hyperpigmentation, which is characterized by dark spots or uneven skin tone brought on by exposure to the sun, inflammation, or hormonal changes, is another common cause for concern. Common indicators of aging include fine lines and wrinkles, which are frequently made worse by environmental stresses including pollution and UV rays.

Furthermore, mild yet efficient treatments are needed for sensitive skin problems like rosacea or eczema to reduce inflammation and fortify the skin barrier. Knowing these frequent worries aids in the selection of suitable sophisticated remedies that precisely target particular problems. A customized strategy may be required for each issue, such as chemical exfoliation for acne, laser therapy for pigmentation correction.

PROFESSIONAL GUIDANCE'S BENEFITS

Without the assistance of a beauty expert, navigating sophisticated skincare procedures can be intimidating. Consulting a specialist guarantees that the treatments are customized to your specific skin type, worries, and objectives. Dermatologists and licensed estheticians are examples of skincare professionals with the knowledge and experience to suggest the best products and treatments based on comprehensive skin evaluations and medical histories.

Furthermore, seeking professional assistance reduces the possibility of negative side effects or other issues resulting from poorly executed therapies. Experts can keep an eye on skin reactions and modify treatment regimens as necessary to maximize outcomes while maintaining patient safety. Additionally, they offer insightful instruction on skincare practices and product suggestions made to preserve and improve treatment results over time. Working with a skincare expert gives people the knowledge and confidence to make decisions about their skincare journey that will lead to healthier, more beautiful skin.

HAVING REASONABLE EXPECTATIONS

When starting advanced skincare treatments, it is important to have reasonable expectations. These treatments are not quick fixes, but they can produce noticeable improvements in the texture, tone, and look of the skin. It's crucial to realize that, depending on how serious the issue is, getting the desired results can take several sessions spread out across time.

Advanced therapies may also cause short-term adverse effects, like redness, slight swelling, or dryness; they are usually brief and go away as the skin recovers. Understanding the gradual nature of skincare changes, the value of patience, and the necessity of adhering to advised post-treatment care routines are all part of setting realistic expectations.

People can confidently navigate their skincare journey by coordinating their expectations with the advice of skincare professionals, understanding that every treatment session contributes to the long-term health and vibrancy of their skin.

CHAPTER TWO

OVERVIEW OF ADVANCED SKINCARE PROCEDURES

THE VALUE OF CUTTING-EDGE THERAPIES

Sophisticated skincare treatments are essential for treating complicated skin issues that may be too difficult for regular skincare regimens to handle. These treatments are intended to address particular problems that call for more involved methods than regular cleansing and moisturizing, such as deep wrinkles, extensive acne scars, hyperpigmentation, and advanced indications of age. Your skin tone, texture, and general appearance can all be significantly and visibly improved by adding sophisticated treatments to your skincare routine.

The capacity of advanced skincare procedures to produce better results than those of basic skincare practices is one of its main advantages. They frequently make use of powerful active ingredients and state-of-the-art technology that reach deeper layers of the skin, encouraging cellular renewal, boosting collagen formation, and mending damage at the cellular level. This focused method addresses underlying problems that regular skincare may not be able to adequately control, improving the skin's appearance while also promoting long-term skin health.

Furthermore, customized advanced skincare treatments are designed to address specific skin types and conditions, guaranteeing an individualized approach to skincare. Whether your skin type is mixed, oily, dry, or sensitive, there are targeted treatments that can successfully address particular issues.

ADVANTAGES OF USING CUTTING-EDGE THERAPIES

Beyond what basic skincare can accomplish, incorporating advanced skincare treatments into your routine offers a multitude of benefits. Because they promote the formation of collagen and elastin, these therapies are quite effective in reversing the obvious indications of aging, such as fine lines, wrinkles, and sagging skin. They can also lessen the appearance of blemishes, scars, and uneven pigmentation for a more even and smoother complexion. They can help improve the texture and tone of the skin.

The capacity of cutting-edge treatments to precisely address particular skin issues is another important advantage. Whether you battle with chronic redness, acne, or sun damage, cutting-edge treatments provide focused solutions that deal with these problems head-on. This focused approach guarantees that you accomplish the intended results more quickly while also accelerating the results.

Furthermore, experienced supervision and knowledge are frequently involved in sophisticated skincare treatments, guaranteeing secure and efficient processes. Experts like qualified estheticians or dermatologists can prescribe and carry out procedures specific to your skin's requirements, guaranteeing the best possible outcomes with the least amount of danger of consequences. You will feel more confident in the treatments you receive with this guidance, which is crucial for navigating the complexities of cutting-edge skincare technologies and chemicals.

THE DISTINCTIONS BETWEEN ADVANCED AND BASIC SKINCARE

To properly treat your skincare difficulties, you must comprehend the distinctions between basic and advanced skincare. Basic skincare usually consists of routines like washing, moisturizing, and protecting the sun. These are vital for preserving the health of the skin and avoiding common problems like UV damage and dryness. These regimens emphasize preserving the skin's natural moisture content and barrier function.

Advanced skincare, on the other hand, targets particular skin disorders with more potent treatments and specialty products than just regular upkeep. To tackle issues like deep wrinkles, acne scars, and uneven pigmentation, advanced skincare treatments may involve chemical peels, microdermabrasion, laser therapy, and advanced facials that reach deeper layers of the skin. For best outcomes, these treatments are customized to each patient's unique skin type and condition, which frequently calls for professional knowledge.

Furthermore, compared to basic skincare formulas, advanced skincare solutions usually contain more concentrated and effective chemicals. Advanced skincare products frequently contain active chemicals like retinoids, alpha hydroxy acids (AHAs), and antioxidants to encourage collagen synthesis, cell turnover, and skin damage healing.

RECOGNIZING SKIN CONDITIONS AND TYPES

To choose the most advanced skincare treatments for your skin type and issues, it is essential to understand them. Different skincare techniques are needed for each type of skin, which can range from oily to dry, sensitive to combination to normal, to achieve balance and health. Assessing elements like oil production, moisture, susceptibility to different products, and environmental conditions are all part of figuring out your skin type.

Apart from determining the kind of skin, pinpointing particular skin issues like acne, rosacea, hyperpigmentation, and indications of aging aids in selecting focused therapies that efficiently tackle these issues. Innovative skincare products are frequently made to address particular ailments by focusing on the root causes of these problems with the use of chemicals and technologies. For example, salicylic acid or benzoyl peroxide are used in acne treatments to clear pores and reduce inflammation; retinoids or peptides are used in anti-aging therapies to stimulate collagen formation and smooth fine wrinkles.

Additionally, speaking with a skincare expert like a dermatologist or certified esthetician can offer insightful advice about the best treatments for your particular skin type. These professionals may perform skin exams, suggest appropriate treatments, and create customized skincare routines that address your issues with the least amount of risk associated with negative reactions or problems.

SAFETY FACTORS FOR COMPLEX THERAPIES

Given the intensity of sophisticated skincare treatments and the potential consequences of improper execution, safety is of the utmost importance. It is crucial to speak with a trained skincare specialist before beginning any advanced treatment. They can determine whether your skin is a good fit for a given technique and make sure you are aware of all the risks and advantages.

For advanced skin care treatments to limit the risk of unpleasant effects, such as allergic reactions, skin irritation, or difficulties after treatment, professional supervision is essential. Professionals in skincare have the know-how to carry out procedures in a safe manner while employing the right techniques and keeping an eye on your skin's reaction to each treatment.

Furthermore, to make well-informed judgments regarding your skincare routine, it's critical to comprehend the technology and substances utilized in sophisticated skincare treatments. To maximize outcomes and reduce discomfort or consequences, many treatments may use chemicals or technologies that call for special precautions or after-treatment care.

You may reap the rewards of cutting-edge skincare treatments while making sure that your skin health is preserved and enhanced for long-term effects by putting safety first and consulting a professional. In addition, under professional supervision, treatment programs can be modified in response to your skin's reaction, guaranteeing that you will safely and successfully attain the intended results.

CHAPTER THREE

CHEMICAL PEELS: SKIN REJUVENATION

CHEMICAL PEELS: WHAT ARE THEY?

Chemical peels are sophisticated skincare procedures that exfoliate the skin by eliminating dead skin cells and encouraging the growth of new, healthy skin. This procedure addresses problems like wrinkles, hyperpigmentation, acne scars, and uneven skin tone, all of which contribute to the skin's improved texture and appearance.

The way the treatment works is that the skin is treated with a chemical solution, which causes the skin to exfoliate and eventually peel off, exposing skin that is smoother and more luminous underneath.

Chemical peels can contain a variety of active agents, but often utilized substances include trichloroacetic acid (TCA), glycolic acid, alpha hydroxy acids (AHAs), and beta hydroxy acids (BHAs) like salicylic acid.

Each of these substances offers a particular level of exfoliation and treatment intensity, focusing on different skin layers. Chemical peels produce a more youthful complexion by increasing cell turnover and stimulating collagen formation by eliminating the outermost layers of damaged skin.

Chemical peels can be customized to address various skin types and issues. They come in different strengths, ranging from mild peels that don't need any downtime to deeper peels that could need more time to heal. Determining the best kind of chemical peel to accomplish your skincare objectives can be aided by knowing the unique requirements of your skin and speaking with a dermatologist.

CHEMICAL PEEL TYPES AVAILABLE

Chemical peels can be broadly classified into three types: medium, deep, and superficial. Superficial peels, also called "lunchtime peels," gently exfoliate the skin's outermost layer using moderate acids like AHAs.

Minor facial defects including fine wrinkles, moderate acne, and uneven skin tone can all be improved with these peels. They are a well-liked option for people leading hectic lives because they demand little downtime.

With the use of stronger acids like TCA, medium peels target deeper layers of the skin. More severe skin conditions such as moderate wrinkles, acne scars, and hyperpigmentation can be effectively treated with them. A medium peel causes more obvious peeling and takes longer to heal, taking a few days to a week for the skin to recuperate and show off its enhanced tone and texture.

The most aggressive type of peels are deep ones, which target the skin's deepest layers with strong chemicals like phenol. Severe skin issues including deep wrinkles, considerable UV damage, and major scarring are appropriate candidates for these peels. Deep peels are intense procedures that need a longer recovery period—often several weeks—and should only be done by trained professionals to reduce hazards and guarantee the best possible outcomes.

HOW TO GET READY FOR A CHEMICAL PEEL

For a chemical peel to be successful and to reduce any possible adverse effects, preparation is essential. It's crucial to speak with a dermatologist before getting a chemical peel to find out which kind is best for your skin type and concerns. To make sure your skin is in the best possible condition before the procedure, they could suggest a pre-peel skincare routine that consists of sunscreen, moisturizers, and gentle cleansers.

It's best to stay away from retinoid-containing treatments, exfoliants, and any other compounds that can irritate the skin in the weeks before the peel. These cosmetics may make the skin more sensitive and raise the possibility of negative responses while peeling. Sun exposure and tanning beds should also be avoided because sunburned or tanned skin is more vulnerable to harm from chemical peels.

Make sure to properly cleanse your skin the day of the peel to get rid of any oils, makeup, and pollutants. Use only the skincare products that your doctor has prescribed. By taking these precautions, you may assist in guaranteeing that your skin is sufficiently ready for the chemical peel, enabling the best possible outcomes and lowering the possibility of issues.

HOW TO DO A CHEMICAL PEEL AT HOME SAFELY

If done properly, using a chemical peel at home can be a safe and efficient technique to get smoother, more youthful-looking skin. To begin, choose a moderate, superficial peel that may be used at home, such as one that contains BHAs or AHAs. To prevent over-exfoliating or injuring your skin, it is imperative that you carefully follow the directions included with the peel product.

To start, give your face a good cleaning to get rid of any debris, oil, or makeup. Spread the chemical peel solution evenly over your face, taking care to avoid getting any in the delicate areas near your mouth and eyes. As directed by the product, let the solution remain on your skin for the prescribed period—typically a few minutes. It's usual to feel a slight tingling or stinging feeling. However, you should quickly rinse the solution off with cool water if you experience severe burning or irritation.

Once the allotted time has passed, neutralize the peel if the product directions call for it, then thoroughly rinse your face with lukewarm water to get rid of any remaining chemical solution.

Using a soft towel, pat dry your skin, then use a light moisturizer to hydrate and calm it. For a few days after the peel, refrain from using any harsh or active skincare products to give your skin time to repair and rejuvenate.

TIPS FOR POST-PEEL SKINCARE

Skincare after peeling must be done properly to provide the best possible outcomes and reduce any possible negative effects. Your skin may be more sensitive, irritable, and red after a chemical peel. It is essential to protect your skin from damaging UV rays and prevent hyperpigmentation by avoiding direct sun exposure and wearing broad-spectrum sunscreen with at least SPF 30 every day, even on overcast days.

It's essential to moisturize your skin frequently to keep it hydrated and aid in the healing process. Apply a light moisturizer that doesn't include any smell to prevent skin irritation.

For at least a week following the peel, stay away from using any skincare products that contain retinoids, acids, or other active chemicals as these might exacerbate irritation and slow the healing process.

You can risk infection or scarring if you scrape or pull at the peeling skin; instead, let it peel and shed naturally. To encourage healing and preserve the health of your skin, use calming and moisturizing products like hyaluronic acid serums or aloe vera gel.

Also, be patient and kind to your skin. Maintaining a glowing, refreshed complexion and getting the most out of your chemical peel are both possible with these post-peel skincare tips.

CHAPTER FOUR

MICRODERMABRASION: A SKIN SMOOTHING PROCEDURE

SYNOPSIS OF MICRODERMABRASION

A non-invasive skincare technique called microdermabrasion aims to smooth and rejuvenate the skin's texture. Because it can treat a variety of skin issues, such as uneven pigmentation, fine lines, wrinkles, and acne scars, this treatment is well-liked. A specialized tool exfoliates the skin's outermost layer during a session, eliminating dead cells and promoting cell turnover. Through this procedure, the skin beneath is made to appear younger and more radiant, resulting in a more even skin tone.

The process can be tailored to each person's unique skin type and issues and is usually carried out by skilled skincare specialists. Microdermabrasion is a versatile solution for anyone wishing to improve the appearance of their skin without downtime or discomfort because it works well on the majority of skin tones and textures. It's crucial to speak with a dermatologist or esthetician to find out if microdermabrasion is the best option for your unique skin care requirements and objectives.

HOW MICRODERMABRASION OPERATES

To delicately abrade the skin's surface, microdermabrasion uses a handheld device that provides a regulated spray of fine crystals or a wand with a diamond tip. The stratum corneum, the skin's outermost layer, is thoroughly cleared of dirt, pollutants, and dead skin cells with this mechanical exfoliation procedure. Over time, tighter, more elastic skin is a result of the device's stimulation of collagen formation and circulation as it glides across the skin.

The process is painless and usually takes between thirty and sixty minutes to finish, depending on the areas that need to be treated and how intensely. During the session, patients may feel a slight scratching or vibrating sensation, although this is usually tolerable.

Similar to moderate sunburn, the skin may appear somewhat reddish or flushed after microdermabrasion; this normally goes away in a few hours to a day.

BENEFITS AND LIMITATIONS OF MICRODERMABRASION

Microdermabrasion offers various benefits, including improving skin texture and tone, reducing the appearance of fine lines and wrinkles, lowering pore size, and boosting the skin's overall luminosity. In addition, it can help reduce hyperpigmentation and acne scars, which makes it a popular option for people looking for non-surgical treatments for common skin care issues. Nevertheless, it's important to remember that deep wrinkles, severe acne, and other skin disorders might not be good candidates for microdermabrasion.

One drawback of microdermabrasion is that it usually takes many weeks between treatments to get the best effects.

Furthermore, before beginning any treatment, people with sensitive skin or those with rosacea should speak with a dermatologist to be sure the course of action is safe and suitable for their skin type. Although most people find microdermabrasion to be safe and effective, individual skin features and compliance with aftercare recommendations can affect the outcome.

GETTING READY FOR A MICRODERMABRASION PROCEDURE

To guarantee the best possible outcome and reduce any possible side effects, there are a few measures involved in getting ready for a microdermabrasion treatment. To find out if you're a good candidate for treatment, it's important to discuss any medications, skincare products, or medical concerns with your skincare provider before your appointment. To minimize excessive skin sensitivity in the days before your visit, avoid using harsh skincare products or exfoliating scrubs.

To ensure that the process is carried out by the practitioner efficiently on the day of your treatment, please arrive with clean, makeup-free skin. Plan a quick appointment to go over your skincare objectives and any last-minute queries or concerns. Dress comfortably. By following these preparatory guidelines, you may increase the overall efficacy of the procedure and guarantee a seamless and successful microdermabrasion experience.

TIPS FOR MAINTENANCE AND AFTERCARE

To get the best results and encourage skin healing following microdermabrasion, you must adhere to certain aftercare guidelines. Use a light moisturizer as soon as possible to replenish moisture and shield the skin from outside influences. To protect the freshly exfoliated skin and prevent sunburn, stay out of direct sunlight and wear sunscreen with an SPF of 30 or higher.

For at least a week following treatment, avoid using abrasive skincare products, chemical peels, or harsh exfoliants to allow the skin to heal correctly. To extend the advantages of microdermabrasion, stay hydrated by drinking lots of water and following a good skincare regimen. Make follow-up sessions as advised by your skincare specialist to preserve the healthiest possible state of your skin and to discuss any queries or concerns that may surface following treatment. Long-term benefits of smoother, more luminous skin can be achieved by following these aftercare recommendations.

CHAPTER FIVE

MICRONEEDLING: IMPROVING THE TEXTURE OF SKIN

COMPREHENDING MICRONEEDLING THERAPY

Collagen induction treatment, another name for microneedling therapy, is a minimally invasive procedure that seeks to improve the texture and renew the skin. Microscopic needles are used to precisely inflict microscopic punctures in the skin's outer layers during microneedling. These tiny cuts encourage the skin's natural healing process and increase the creation of elastin and collagen. As a result, throughout time, the texture of the skin gets more even, firm, and smooth.

To reduce discomfort, the area is first cleaned and a numbing lotion is applied. The treatment area is then gently rolled or pressed over a microneedling device, which can be a derma roller or a pen-like instrument with fine needles.

The particular skin issues being addressed, such as fine lines, wrinkles, acne scars, or uneven skin tone, determine how deeply the needle penetrates the skin. Following the procedure, the skin could look a little reddish or puffy, similar to a little sunburn, but this usually goes away in a day or two.

Microneedling is helpful for diverse skin types and can be tailored based on individual needs. To get the best benefits, it is advised to have numerous sessions spaced a few weeks apart. All things considered, microneedling is a flexible procedure that uses the body's healing processes to improve the texture and renewal of the skin.

MICRONEEDLING DEVICE TYPES

There are various types of micro needling devices, each intended to target a certain skincare issue and produce the best possible outcomes. Derma rollers and microneedling pens are the two main categories of microneedling equipment. With a derma roller, hundreds of microscopic needles are embedded in a cylindrical roller that is manually rolled over the skin to produce microchannels. Longer needles are more suited for deeper penetration, whereas shorter needles are better for treatments that are applied superficially on these rollers.

Conversely, an automated tool with adjustable needle depths is used in microneedling pens, such as the well-known Dermapen. These pens are perfect for targeting specific skin conditions like fine lines and acne scars since they produce precise and controlled needle penetrations at the right depth and pace. The consistent and even covering of the treated areas is guaranteed by the automated movement of the microneedling pens.

Derma rollers and microneedling pens both increase the formation of collagen and improve the absorption of products; however, pens are more precise and are frequently used in professional treatments. The intended treatment depth, skin sensitivity, and the skill of the practitioner executing the process all play a role in selecting the best microneedling tool.

MICRO NEEDLING'S BENEFITS FOR SKIN REJUVENATION

Microneedling is a popular option for people who want to improve the texture and appearance of their skin because it provides several advantages for skin renewal. Collagen induction—a process whereby the micro-injuries made during the operation promote the development of collagen and elastin—is one of the main advantages. Over time, this results in skin that is smoother, firmer, and has fewer wrinkles and fine lines.

Additionally, by lessening the visibility of scars, such as surgical and acne scars, microneedling helps to improve the texture of the skin. The micro-channels that the needles generate also improve skincare products' absorption and efficacy by facilitating improved diffusion of active substances into the skin's deeper layers. When applied in conjunction with microneedling, this can enhance the advantages of serums, moisturizers, and other topical therapies.

The adaptability of microneedling in treating a range of skin issues, including hyperpigmentation, uneven skin tone, and enlarged pores, is another noteworthy benefit. The majority of patients had moderate redness and swelling following the minimally invasive surgery, which usually goes away in a few days. All things considered, microneedling is a non-surgical way to get skin that is smoother, more radiant, and has long-lasting effects.

GETTING READY FOR NEEDLING ON YOUR SKIN

It is essential to properly prepare your skin before a microneedling session to maximize outcomes and reduce the possibility of problems. To establish the best course of action for treating your skin type, start by speaking with a skincare expert. To avoid skin sensitivity and irritation, it is imperative to stop using several skincare products, like retinoids and exfoliating acids, at least one week before microneedling.

Make sure to thoroughly cleanse your skin the day of your consultation to get rid of any oil, debris, or makeup residue. A spotless canvas lowers the possibility of bacterial contamination and enhances the effectiveness of the microneedling device's skin penetration. Use a numbing cream on the treatment region as directed by your practitioner to reduce pain during the process.

Maintaining proper hydration and limiting sun exposure in the days preceding microneedling are also crucial. Skin that is too sensitive or sunburned may not respond well to therapy and may have negative side effects. You may contribute to ensuring a safe and effective microneedling procedure that optimizes the benefits of skin rejuvenation by adhering to these pre-treatment suggestions.

AFTER-TREATMENT CARE AND MONITORING

Adequate aftercare is necessary to optimize the healing process and improve the outcomes of microneedling therapy. Your skin may seem red and feel a little sensitive just after treatment, much like small sunburn. This is common and goes away in a few hours to a day, depending on how intensive the therapy is.

To ensure that the skin heals properly, stay away from putting makeup or other skincare products in the treated region for at least 24 hours. To hydrate the skin and aid with healing, your practitioner can advise using a mild cleanser and moisturizer. To prevent UV damage to the skin that has been treated, it is imperative to stay out of the direct sun and to use sunscreen with an SPF of at least thirty.

As the skin goes through its natural renewal process, you can see some peeling or flaking in the days after microneedling. To avoid scarring and to let the old skin layers fall off naturally, refrain from scraping or scratching the skin. To reduce the chance of irritation, adhere to any extra post-care recommendations made by your skincare specialist, such as staying away from saunas and strenuous exercise.

As advised by your practitioner, arrange follow-up appointments to preserve and improve the effects of microneedling. It could take multiple treatments separated by a few weeks to get the desired improvements in the texture and look of the skin. You may enjoy smoother, healthier-looking skin for a longer period by following a thorough post-treatment regimen and scheduling follow-up consultations.

CHAPTER SIX

LASER THERAPY: FOCUSING ON SKIN CONCERNS

OVERVIEW OF LASER SKINCARE PROCEDURES

The way we treat a variety of skin issues has changed dramatically because of laser skincare procedures, which provide accurate, long-lasting remedies with little recovery time. Concentrated laser beams are used in these treatments to target particular skin conditions like wrinkles, pigmentation, acne scars, and even unwanted hair. For novices hoping to enhance the appearance and health of their skin, knowing the fundamentals of laser treatments is essential.

For laser treatments to be effective, precise light pulses must be delivered to the skin. There, the targeted tissue must absorb the light pulses. Over time, this process promotes skin cell renewal and collagen formation, giving the skin a smoother, more even tone. People who are new to laser skincare must speak with a licensed dermatologist or skincare specialist to figure out the best course of action depending on their skin type, issues, and desired results.

Beyond only improving appearance, laser treatments can also successfully treat medical disorders including vascular lesions and rosacea. It's crucial to approach these treatments, therefore, with reasonable expectations and comprehension of the associated procedure. Beginners can easily traverse the world of laser skincare treatments with the right advice and preparation, knowing they are moving toward healthier, more youthful skin.

KINDS OF LASER THERAPY OFFERED

There are multiple varieties of laser therapies, each intended to target particular skin issues and ailments. For example, ablative lasers, including CO2 and Erbium YAG lasers, work well to repair deep wrinkles and scars because they remove the outer layers of skin and increase the formation of collagen. Non-destructive lasers, such as Nd

and Alexandrite lasers, which target pigmentation problems and promote tissue tightness without harming the skin's outer layer, function underneath the surface of the skin.

Fractional lasers, like Fraxel and Pixel lasers, use precise energy microbeams to inflict microscopic lesions on the skin, which prompt the body's natural healing process and encourage the creation of new tissue. With little downtime, these procedures are great for decreasing pore size, smoothing out fine wrinkles, and enhancing skin texture. Furthermore, by precisely targeting hair follicles, diode or alexandrite laser hair removal treatments provide a long-term cure for unwanted hair.

The kind of skin, the severity of the ailment being treated, and the intended results all play a role in selecting the best laser treatment. To find out which kind of laser therapy will best help them reach their skincare objectives, beginners should speak with a licensed dermatologist or skincare specialist. Comprehending the distinctions among these therapies enables people to make knowledgeable choices regarding their skincare routine, guaranteeing secure and efficient outcomes.

SAFETY ISSUES REGARDING LASER TREATMENTS

Although laser treatments are usually safe and effective when administered by qualified specialists, there are a few crucial safety factors to be aware of. To reduce the chance of issues, selecting a trustworthy facility or provider with laser skincare experience is crucial. A comprehensive consultation should be held to determine skin type, medical history, and potential dangers before receiving any laser therapy.

Beginners should be aware that adverse effects from laser treatments, such as redness, swelling, or slight discomfort, are possible but usually go away in a few days. Optimizing recovery and results can be achieved by adhering to post-treatment care guidelines, which include minimizing sun exposure and using suggested skincare products.

Furthermore, particular laser settings could be necessary for those with darker skin tones or certain medical problems to reduce the possibility of pigmentation changes or other negative consequences.

Protection eyewear is usually provided before each laser session to protect the eyes from the powerful light that is released during treatment. To make sure they have a comfortable and safe experience, patients should discuss any worries or inquiries they may have with their clinician.

GETTING READY FOR LASER THERAPY SESSIONS

To guarantee the best possible outcome and reduce any possible side effects, there are a few measures involved in getting ready for laser treatment sessions.

It's crucial to adhere to any pre-treatment guidelines given by the skincare expert or clinic before the consultation. This can entail staying away from specific skincare products, drugs, or activities that might aggravate skin irritation or impair the laser's efficiency.

It is best to arrive on the day of the treatment with clean, makeup-free skin to enable a complete evaluation and setup. To improve comfort during the process, numbing cream may be administered to the treatment region, depending on the type of laser treatment that is planned. To prevent negative reactions, patients should inform their clinician in advance of any allergies or sensitivities.

To promote skin healing and recovery, it is essential to be hydrated before and after laser treatments. Water consumption can affect the skin's reaction to laser therapy by preserving skin suppleness and general moisture levels. On the day of treatment, it can also help to prevent irritation and facilitate easy access to the treatment region by dressing comfortably and loosely.

Beginners can maximize their laser therapy experience and help achieve desired skincare benefits by following these pre-treatment measures. A seamless procedure is ensured, and laser skincare treatments are more successful when there is open communication with the treatment provider and adherence to pre-treatment instructions.

CONTROLLING RESULTS AND EXPECTATIONS

Undergoing laser skincare treatments requires managing expectations and comprehending realistic outcomes. Although skin texture, tone, and clarity can be greatly improved with these treatments, each person will experience improvement to a different degree. Results can be influenced by variables like age, skin type, and the severity of the ailment being treated.

After a series of laser treatments spaced several weeks apart, the skin usually heals and regenerates in between treatments before substantial benefits become apparent. Beginners should approach laser skincare cautiously because it may take several months for the desired effects to become apparent. It's common to have transient adverse effects during the healing process, such as redness or light peeling, but they should go away as the skin recovers.

Skincare experts frequently advise a customized skincare routine that consists of moisturizers, mild cleansers, and sunscreen to prevent sun damage to the skin to preserve and improve results. It is possible to arrange for routine follow-up sessions to assess treatment plans and make necessary adjustments. Beginners can see long-lasting benefits in the appearance and general health of their skin by setting reasonable expectations and following post-treatment care instructions.

CHAPTER SEVEN

CUTTING EDGE ANTI-AGING INTERVENTIONS

TYPICAL INDICATIONS OF SKIN CHANGES AND AGING

Our skin changes throughout time in several ways that are frequently noticeable and can impact how we look. Age spots, drooping skin, fine lines, and wrinkles are typical indicators of aging. Several causes, including decreased production of collagen and elastin, a decrease in the turnover of skin cells, and environmental damage from sun exposure, contribute to these changes. Selecting the best anti-aging medicines requires an understanding of these indicators.

Treatments like retinoids and peptides are useful for treating wrinkles and fine lines because they improve skin texture and increase the formation of collagen. Procedures like radiofrequency or laser therapy, which tighten and firm the skin by promoting the formation of collagen and elastin, can be used to cure sagging skin. Ingredients that lighten pigmentation and even out skin tone, like hydroquinone or vitamin C, can help decrease age spots that result from sun exposure.

All things considered, by identifying these indicators, people can successfully customize their skincare regimen to address certain age concerns. The skin might appear smoother, firmer, and younger by selecting the right therapies and comprehending the underlying problems.

AN OVERVIEW OF TREATMENTS FOR ANTI-AGING

The term "anti-aging treatments" refers to a broad category of operations and goods intended to minimize the look of aging on the skin. These treatments can be divided into more intrusive procedures like chemical peels, microdermabrasion, and cosmetic surgery like facelifts or botox injections, as well as non-invasive choices including topical creams, serums, and masks.

Active components found in topical treatments include retinoids, hyaluronic acid, vitamin C, and peptides; these compounds address particular signs of aging, such as wrinkles, loss of elasticity, and uneven skin tone. Chemical peels and other non-invasive procedures exfoliate the skin to expose younger, smoother skin beneath, while microdermabrasion eliminates dead skin cells and encourages the creation of collagen.

If more sophisticated procedures are being considered, facelifts and botox injections can produce impressive results by tightening and raising drooping skin and minimizing the visibility of deep wrinkles. The best course of action should always be determined in consultation with a dermatologist or skincare specialist, taking into account each patient's unique skin type, problems, and desired results.

INGREDIENTS TO CONSIDER IN PRODUCTS TO PREVENT AGING

Knowing important ingredients to look for in anti-aging treatments will help you achieve the results you want. Retinoids, like retinol or tretinoin, are frequently used as effective components because they encourage the creation of collagen and cell turnover, which gradually reduces wrinkles and improves the texture of the skin. Another helpful component is hyaluronic acid, which plumps the face and minimizes the appearance of fine wrinkles due to its moisturizing qualities.

While peptides aid in the stimulation of collagen formation, which improves skin firmness and elasticity, vitamin C is a potent antioxidant that brightens the skin and shields it from environmental damage. Additionally beneficial for lowering inflammation and enhancing skin barrier function, niacinamide (vitamin B3) can also improve the general health and appearance of the skin.

Selecting anti-aging products that contain these components might help your program work better by treating particular issues like wrinkles, dryness, and uneven skin tone. You may noticeably improve the texture, tone, and overall youthfulness of your skin by including these substances in a daily skincare routine that is customized for your skin type and needs.

FACTORS OF LIFESTYLE THAT AFFECT SKIN AGING

Skin aging is largely influenced by lifestyle factors, in addition to skincare products and treatments. One of the main factors contributing to early aging is sun exposure, which produces wrinkles, sunspots, and elasticity loss. Younger skin can be preserved and further damage can be avoided by using sunscreen and avoiding sun exposure.

A diet high in vitamins and antioxidants can support skin health and collagen formation, but some lifestyle choices, like smoking, can hasten the aging process by decreasing blood supply to the skin and resulting in wrinkles. It's also critical to drink enough water since it keeps skin supple and plump.

Controlling stress levels is also important because long-term stress can hasten aging and cause inflammation. Stress-relieving practices like yoga, meditation, and regular exercise can improve general well-being and maintain healthy skin.

Together with skincare treatments, addressing these lifestyle variables helps people maximize their anti-aging efforts and keep their youthful appearance for longer.

DEVELOPING A CUSTOMIZED ANTI-AGING SKINCARE PROGRAM

Understanding each person's unique skin issues, preferences, and goals is essential to creating a customized anti-aging skincare routine. Determine your main concerns with aging, such as wrinkles, dryness, or uneven skin tone, and then choose products and treatments that address those particular problems.

A gentle cleanser to remove pollutants without removing natural oils is usually the first step in a basic regimen. A toner is next used to balance pH levels and prepare the skin for treatment products. Using a serum that is enhanced with active components, such as hyaluronic acid or retinoids, can help with certain issues like dehydration or fine wrinkles.

Especially for aging skin that is prone to dryness, moisturizers are crucial for preserving skin barrier function and retaining moisture.

Select a moisturizer that has been enriched with peptides or antioxidants to offer extra anti-aging advantages and shield the skin from external aggressors.

Using broad-spectrum SPF sunscreen is essential all year round to avoid UV damage and early aging. Even on overcast days or inside, apply sunscreen as the final step in your morning routine to protect your skin from UV radiation.

Finally, to encourage cell turnover and show smoother, more youthful-looking skin, think about incorporating treatments like an enzyme mask or monthly exfoliation with a mild scrub. Adapt your routine as necessary to seasonal variations, skin responses, or any particular issues that may develop over time.

You may successfully treat aging issues and preserve healthy, youthful-looking skin for years to come by adhering to a customized skincare regimen made to fit your specific needs and preferences.

CHAPTER EIGHT

EXPERT FACIAL PROCEDURES: REJUVENATION METHODS

ADVANTAGES OF EXPERT FACIALS

Numerous advantages of professional facials can greatly enhance your skin's appearance and health. First of all, they offer deeper cleansing than is possible with regular at-home regimens. With this deep cleaning, the skin appears clearer and more vibrant while also reducing acne and unclogging pores. Professional facials also frequently incorporate exfoliating methods that remove dead skin cells from the skin, encouraging cell renewal and enhancing skin tone and texture.

The customized care you get from a professional face is another important advantage. Estheticians determine your skin type and target concerns before customizing a facial to meet your requirements. This personalization can guarantee that your skin gets the right care by incorporating anti-aging, hydration, or acne management therapies. The efficacy of facials is further increased by the use of premium, professional-grade products, which provide nutrients and substances that deeply nourish and revitalize the skin.

Professional facials also offer a soothing and therapeutic experience that enhances general well-being. During a facial, massage techniques are employed to stimulate lymphatic drainage and blood circulation, which can help minimize puffiness and give the appearance of healthy skin. Stress levels are also lowered by the experienced touch and calming surroundings, which promotes both physical and mental relaxation.

Therefore, getting a professional facial regularly not only improves the condition of your skin but also gives you a much-needed vacation from the daily grind, which helps you feel more balanced and refreshed.

VARIOUS FACE TREATMENT METHODS

Numerous face treatments are available, each with a unique goal of addressing a particular skin condition and providing desired results. Traditional facials are a favorite because they provide a thorough treatment that includes cleansing, exfoliation, extraction, massage, and a skin-type-specific mask. All skin types can benefit from these facials, which leave the complexion balanced and revitalized.

Chemical peels are a fantastic alternative for people looking for a more extensive course of treatment. Through the application of acids to exfoliate the skin's surface, these treatments help to improve conditions including fine lines, acne scars, and hyperpigmentation by encouraging cell turnover. While downtime may vary depending on the severity of the peel, smoother, more even-toned skin is frequently the outcome. Another cutting-edge procedure is microdermabrasion, which minimizes downtime by using a device to exfoliate the skin's outer layer and efficiently reduce the appearance of wrinkles, UV damage, and enlarged pores.

Specialized facials address certain concerns, such as acne control or anti-aging. Hyaluronic acid, peptides, and antioxidants are examples of substances that anti-aging facials may include to promote the formation of collagen and lessen the visibility of wrinkles. Deep cleaning, extractions, and antimicrobial treatments are frequently used in acne facials to help treat current outbreaks and stop new ones. With so many possibilities, speaking with an esthetician can help you choose the facial treatment that best suits the needs of your skin.

SELECTING THE PROPER FACIAL BASED ON YOUR SKIN TYPE

To get the best results, choose the facial that is best for your skin type. Hydrating facials are advised for people with dry skin. With an emphasis on restoring moisture levels, these facials frequently contain hyaluronic acid, aloe vera, and soothing oils. The intention is to moisturize and calm the skin, leaving it feeling dewy and silky. Facials with abrasive exfoliants or alcohol-based products should be avoided by those with dry skin types because they can make their dryness and irritation worse.

Treatments for oily or acne-prone skin can help reduce excessive oil production and prevent outbreaks. Acne flare-ups are less likely when deep-cleaning facials with extractions help to clear debris and unclog pores. Because of their antibacterial qualities, ingredients like salicylic acid and tea tree oil are frequently utilized. Without overhydrating or overdrying any one part of the face, a tailored strategy that targets both oily and dry areas can help balance the complexion in those with mixed skin.

Gentle treatments are necessary for sensitive skin to prevent irritation and redness. Cucumber, oatmeal, and chamomile are examples of calming components that can be used in calming facials to build the skin's barrier and lessen inflammation. It's critical to let the esthetician know about any allergies or sensitivities in advance so they can adjust the treatment. You may determine your skin type and select the best face treatment to improve the appearance and health of your skin by speaking with a specialist.

WHEN AND HOW OFTEN TO GET FACIAL TREATMENTS

The sort of facial being done and the needs of each individual's skin determine how often and when to get facial treatments. A professional facial is advised every four to six weeks for most skin types. This gives the skin enough time to go through its normal regeneration cycle and enables the treatment of any possible breakouts or problems. Frequent facials provide continual improvement in skin tone and texture as well as skin health by keeping pores clear.

Those with certain skin conditions, including acne or hyperpigmentation, may initially require more regular treatments. For instance, biweekly facials may be beneficial for someone receiving acne treatments until their skin begins to clean up. Reduce the frequency to a maintenance schedule once the condition is under control. It's critical to heed your esthetician's advice regarding the best course of action for your particular skin type and issues.

Scheduling your facials around important occasions can also improve outcomes. It's best to schedule a facial at least a week in advance of important events like weddings or vacations. This makes sure your skin looks its best by allowing any redness or irritation from the treatment to go away. Additionally, as stress can have a detrimental effect on skin health, scheduling facials at less stressful times might optimize the advantages.

IMPROVING OUTCOMES WITH HOMECARE METHODS

Maintaining the advantages in between treatments requires enhancing the results of expert facials with homecare procedures. The benefits of a facial can be prolonged with a regular skincare regimen catered to your specific skin type.

This usually includes daily use of sunscreen, washing, toning, and moisturizing. By following your esthetician's recommendations, you can be confident the products address your unique skin concerns and work in harmony with the expert treatments.

At-home exfoliation is yet another essential method for preserving skin health. Gently exfoliating the skin once or twice a week encourages cell turnover and keeps pores from getting clogged by removing dead skin cells. Take care not to over-exfoliate since this might damage the skin's protective layer and cause irritation. Depending on the components of the mask, adding a weekly face mask can also offer other advantages like hydration, brightness, or detoxification.

Skin health is influenced by eating a balanced diet and drinking plenty of water. In addition to providing vital nutrients, a balanced diet full of fruits, vegetables, and healthy fats keeps the skin hydrated from the inside out.

CHAPTER NINE

TREATMENTS FOR ACNE: RESOLVING SKIN ISSUES

KNOWING THE TYPES AND CAUSES OF ACNE

Several things can lead to acne, such as germs, inflammation, clogged hair follicles, and excessive oil production. Hormonal fluctuations can cause increased oil production and clogged pores, especially during puberty, menstruation, and stressful times. In addition, nutrition, heredity, and some drugs all have a big impact on acne development. Comprehending these reasons is essential for efficient therapy, since tackling the underlying cause aids in choosing the best acne control strategy.

Numerous treatment approaches are needed for the numerous ways that acne presents itself. Blackheads, whiteheads, papules, pustules, nodules, and cysts are among the most prevalent varieties. Called comedonal acne, blackheads and whiteheads are noninflammatory pimples that appear as a result of clogged hair follicles. While nodules and cysts are severe forms of acne that frequently leave scars if not treated appropriately, pustules and papules are red, inflammatory, and occasionally painful. Knowing these kinds helps you tailor skincare regimens and select the right remedies.

For novices, the first step to efficient therapy is determining the precise type of acne. Acne can be prevented from getting worse with simple skincare routines including gentle cleaning, non-comedogenic product use, and avoiding abrasive scrubs. It is imperative to see a dermatologist if acne is severe or persistent since they may offer specialized treatments and advice based on each patient's unique skin requirements. Comprehending the complexities of acne types and reasons enables people to make knowledgeable judgments regarding their skincare regimen.

AN OVERVIEW OF AVAILABLE ACNE TREATMENTS

Options for treating acne include prescription drugs, over-the-counter treatments, and cutting-edge dermatological procedures. Topical medications are frequently used to stimulate cell turnover, clear pores, and reduce inflammation. Examples of these medications include retinoids, salicylic acid, and benzoyl peroxide.

Dermatologists may recommend oral drugs, such as isotretinoin, antibiotics, and hormonal therapy like birth control pills, for patients with moderate to severe acne. These medications target the underlying causes of acne.

Deeper-targeting advanced therapies for acne include chemical peels, laser therapy, and light-based procedures. Acids are used in chemical peels to exfoliate the skin, lower inflammation, and stop breakouts in the future. Blue light and pulsed light therapies, among others, eliminate acne-causing bacteria and lower oil production. Dermatologists usually provide these treatments, which need several sessions to yield the best results.

Acne management also involves the use of natural and alternative therapies. Tea tree oil, aloe vera, and green tea extract are examples of ingredients with anti-inflammatory and antibacterial qualities that offer a more gentle method of treating acne. Acne can also be controlled by dietary changes, such as cutting back on sugar and consuming more omega-3 fatty acids. By looking into these possibilities, people can select the most appropriate and successful course of action for their particular skin issues.

HOME VS. PROFESSIONAL TREATMENTS FOR ACNE

Professional acne treatments from dermatologists or certified skincare specialists are more accurate and effective. These consist of extractions, microdermabrasion, laser therapy, and chemical peels. Acids are applied to the skin during chemical peels to exfoliate, unclog pores, and increase collagen synthesis. By focusing on the deeper layers of the skin, laser and light therapies can reduce inflammation and eradicate germs that cause acne. Through the use of a mechanical tool, microdermabrasion exfoliates the skin, encouraging cell turnover and eliminating dead skin cells. Expert extractions that are carried out with sterile instruments safely remove comedones and minimize scarring.

For mild to moderate acne, at-home treatments are more accessible and can be successful. Breakouts can be controlled with over-the-counter medications that contain alpha hydroxy acids, salicylic acid, and benzoyl peroxide. It's crucial to have a regular skincare regimen that includes moisturizing, protecting the skin from the sun, and mild washing. DIY remedies with anti-inflammatory and antibacterial properties include green tea compresses and honey masks. However, since these methods might make acne worse, it's crucial to stay away from harsh substances and vigorous scrubbing.

Depending on the severity of acne and personal preferences, one can choose between home and expert treatments. Results from professional treatments are more noticeable and faster, especially for severe or chronic acne. For continuous maintenance and minor acne care, at-home treatments are affordable and practical. Under the supervision of a dermatologist, combining the two methods can result in comprehensive treatment and the best possible results.

TAKING CARE OF HYPERPIGMENTATION AND ACNE SCARS

Severe acne frequently leaves hyperpigmentation and scarring on the skin, which can be improved with specialized therapies. Scars and discoloration on the surface can be effectively reduced using chemical peels and microdcrmabrasion. Chemical peels encourage the growth of new, healthier skin by using acids to exfoliate the top layers of the skin. Skin tone and texture are improved by mechanically exfoliating the skin with microdermabrasion. Dermatologists administer these treatments, which usually take several sessions to yield noticeable effects.

For deeper scars and pigmentation problems, advanced laser treatments including intense pulsed light (IPL) and fractional laser therapy are available. Fractional lasers improve skin texture and stimulate the creation of collagen by targeting deeper layers of the skin. Broad-spectrum light is used in IPL to improve skin tone generally and remove pigmentation. For persistent scarring and discoloration, both treatments yield significant benefits, but they also require professional competence and may require considerable downtime.

Topical therapies for pigmentation and post-acne marks include hydroquinone, vitamin C, and retinoids. Retinoids lessen the visibility of scars by accelerating cell turnover and encouraging the synthesis of collagen. Antioxidant vitamin C lightens skin tone and lessens hyperpigmentation. One powerful skin-lightening drug that targets dark spots is hydroquinone. When these therapies are used consistently along with sun protection, acne scars, and hyperpigmentation can be gradually reduced in appearance.

LONG-TERM ACNE PREVENTION TECHNIQUES

Effective skincare techniques, alterations to one's lifestyle, and, when required, medical procedures are all part of long-term acne prevention. It is essential to follow a regular skincare regimen that is customized for each kind of skin. This entails using non-comedogenic moisturizers, cleaning gently, and combining retinoids and salicylic acid—two substances that combat acne. Frequent exfoliation aids in preventing clogged pores, and sun protection reduces hyperpigmentation and inflammation.

Diet and way of living are important factors in acne prevention. Managing acne can be achieved by consuming fewer dairy products, processed sweets, and high-glycemic foods. Overall skin health is supported by incorporating a balanced diet high in fruits, vegetables, lean proteins, and omega-3 fatty acids. Clearer skin is also a result of drinking enough water, getting enough sleep, and using stress-reduction techniques like yoga or meditation. Frequent exercise improves blood flow and lowers stress, two factors that are beneficial to the health of the skin.

Continual dermatological consultation is crucial for people with acne that doesn't go away. They can offer tailored guidance and modify treatments as necessary. Long-term usage of topical or oral medicines, under professional care, may be necessary for controlling chronic acne. Frequent consultations with a skincare specialist guarantee that the tactics selected continue to work and enable prompt modifications.

CHAPTER TEN

TREATMENTS FOR SKIN BRIGHTENING: ATTAINING RADIANCE

OVERVIEW OF SKIN BRIGHTENING METHODS

By minimizing dark spots, enhancing overall skin tone, and encouraging a more radiant complexion, skin lightening procedures seek to increase skin radiance. These methods are very popular for treating skin tone irregularities, dullness, and hyperpigmentation brought on by aging, sun exposure, and hormone changes. Using topical medications that increase skin cell turnover and target melanin formation is one of the most popular approaches.

Alpha hydroxy acids (AHAs), niacinamide, and vitamin C are common constituents in these treatments; they all act together to brighten and revitalize the skin.

Furthermore, more aggressive methods of skin lightening are provided by procedures like chemical peels and laser treatments, which successfully target the skin's deeper layers to minimize pigmentation and increase the formation of collagen. Different skin types and issues are catered to by the varying intensities and outcomes of each treatment. To get brighter and more radiant skin, it's critical to comprehend the unique needs of your skin and speak with a dermatologist or skincare specialist to identify the best course of action.

TREATMENTS FOR SKIN BRIGHTENING: TYPES

There are many different types of skin-lightening treatments available, ranging from mild everyday routines to more involved clinical procedures. Brightening serums and creams with components like retinoids, licorice extract, and kojic acid—which help prevent the formation of melanin and encourage skin renewal—are frequently a part of everyday skincare regimes.

Regular application of these items helps to progressively lessen dark spots and enhance the general clarity of the skin.

Professional procedures like chemical peels and microdermabrasion, which efficiently remove dead skin cells and promote cell turnover, provide deeper levels of exfoliation for those looking for quicker results. Chemical peels remove the outer layer of skin to expose smoother, more vibrant skin beneath by using acids like salicylic acid or glycolic acid. In contrast, laser treatments use high-energy light to specifically target pigmented regions to break down melanin deposits and stimulate the creation of collagen, giving the appearance of more young and even-toned skin.

The best skin-brightening therapy depends on several criteria, including skin sensitivity, desired results, and financial constraints. To guarantee safety and efficacy, these procedures must be carried out under the guidance of a licensed skincare specialist.

COMPONENTS FOR EVEN SKIN TONE AND BRIGHTENING

Using strong substances that can lessen hyperpigmentation and encourage a more even skin tone is essential for effective skin lightening. Strong antioxidant vitamin C prevents the synthesis of melanin and lightens skin by scavenging free radicals from UV exposure. In the long run, it improves skin elasticity and texture by increasing the manufacture of collagen.

Niacinamide, a type of vitamin B3, is good for oily and acne-prone skin because it reduces dark spots and regulates sebum production when combined with vitamin C.

Glycolic acid and lactic acid are examples of alpha hydroxy acids (AHAs) that gently exfoliate the skin to remove dead cells and reveal brighter skin underneath. Additionally, by increasing cell turnover, these acids lessen the visibility of wrinkles and fine lines.

Additional advantageous components consist of licorice extract, which helps lighten black spots and has anti-inflammatory qualities, and kojic acid, which is produced from mushrooms and has skin-lightening capabilities. These components work together in skincare products to target several phases of melanin formation and offer complete brightening benefits for a more radiant face.

RISKS AND PRECAUTIONS RELATED TO BRIGHTENING TREATMENTS

Although skin-brightening therapies have the potential to yield remarkable outcomes, improper usage of these treatments may result in dangers and adverse effects. Temporary redness, dryness, or increased sensitivity to sunlight is common side effects, particularly after treatments like chemical peels and laser therapy. To reduce these dangers and optimize results, it's critical to adhere to your dermatologist's post-treatment care instructions.

Certain compounds found in brightening solutions, such as AHAs and retinoids, can irritate sensitive people or trigger allergic responses. It is advised to patch-test new products before complete use to determine skin tolerance and avoid negative reactions. Furthermore, people with darker skin tones should use caution while undergoing intense lightening procedures because they may be more vulnerable to post-inflammatory hyperpigmentation (PIH).

Before beginning any brightening routine, it is imperative to speak with a dermatologist or skincare specialist to assess your skin type, address any issues, and choose the safest and most efficient course of action for attaining more even-toned, brighter skin.

INCLUDING TREATMENTS FOR BRIGHTENING SKIN IN YOUR SKINCARE ROUTINE

When applied appropriately and consistently, skin-lightening treatments can improve the overall health and appearance of your skin. Apply a brightening serum or treatment with components like vitamin C or niacinamide after washing your face gently with a cleanser that is appropriate for your skin type. Over time, these products assist to even out skin tone and target dark areas.

Using a gentle exfoliant, like a scrub or an enzyme-based mask, as part of your weekly routine will assist in removing dead skin cells and encourage cell turnover. By going deeper into the skin, this step increases the efficacy of the skincare products that follow.

Every few months, think about adding in-office procedures like chemical peels or microdermabrasion to your skincare routine for better outcomes. Smoother, more radiant skin is revealed with these treatments, which target persistent pigmentation and deliver a deeper exfoliation.

To protect your skin from UV rays and stop hyperpigmented spots from getting darker, apply a broad-spectrum sunscreen with SPF 30 or higher afterward. When including brightening treatments into your skincare routine, consistency and patience are essential because continuous use along with appropriate sun protection can lead to a gradual improvement in skin tone and clarity.

CHAPTER ELEVEN
SELECTING THE BEST SKINCARE EXPERT

CHARACTERISTICS OF A SKINCARE EXPERT

A trustworthy skincare expert should have completed a rigorous school program in dermatology or esthetics to guarantee they have the fundamental understanding needed for more complex procedures. This entails knowing the different types of skin disorders, their anatomy, and the newest advancements in skincare technology. Certification from an accredited college and proof of continued education is important to look for because skincare is a sector that is always changing with new methods and products.

Another essential component is experience. A skilled skincare specialist has a history of pleasing customers and effective treatments. They ought to be ready to offer client endorsements in addition to before and after pictures of their job. Their hands-on training enables them to efficiently handle unforeseen responses or complications and customize therapies to meet the needs of each patient.

The importance of interpersonal skills is equal. A competent skin care specialist should be kind, pay close attention to your worries, and explain methods and anticipated results in plain language. They ought to create a welcoming and trustworthy atmosphere that will boost your self-assurance and ease you on your skincare path. A top-tier specialist will demonstrate professionalism, sensitivity, and a sincere desire to assist you in reaching your skincare objectives.

FINDING AND CHOOSING A SKINCARE EXPERT

Obtain suggestions from dependable people, such as friends, family, or medical professionals, to begin your quest. An expert's reputation and client satisfaction can also be discerned through online reviews and ratings on sites like Yelp and Google. Seek out recurrently positive reviews and take notice of any issues that are brought up again and again.

Verify the specialist's qualifications to execute advanced skincare treatments by looking through their credentials and certificates. Check if they are members of any professional associations, including the International Society of Aesthetic Plastic Surgery (ISAPS) or the American Academy of Dermatology (AAD). These affiliations frequently signify a dedication to high standards and continuing education for professionals.

To learn more about the specialist's experience and the spectrum of therapies they provide, visit their website and social media accounts. Search for thorough process explanations, informative blog entries, and customer endorsements. This can provide you with an overview of their practice and assist you in determining whether their methodology is in line with your skincare objectives and demands.

THINGS TO BRING UP IN YOUR CONSULTATION

Inquire about the skincare specialist's experience with the particular treatments you are considering when you meet with them for a consultation. Find out how often they have completed these surgeries and ask to view before and after pictures of previous patients. This will help you gauge their level of expertise and the kind of outcomes you should anticipate.

Talk to the specialist about your aims and concerns regarding skincare in detail, and ask them to clarify the suggested course of action. Ascertain that they clearly outline the steps that will solve your particular problems, the anticipated time frame for completion, and any possible negative impacts or downtime. This openness sets reasonable expectations and aids in decision-making.

Inquire about follow-up and post-treatment care. It is essential to comprehend the aftercare guidelines and any required follow-up consultations to preserve your outcomes and guarantee appropriate skin healing. Throughout your treatment process, a competent skin care specialist will provide thorough advice and support, stressing the value of continued care and routine check-ins.

ASSESSING RECOMMENDATIONS AND TREATMENT PLANS

Make sure the skincare specialist's recommended course of action fits both your skin type and your goals by carefully going over it. A customized plan should be created, taking into consideration your lifestyle, medical history, and particular skin concerns. Generic plans or cookie-cutter are a warning sign because sophisticated skincare treatments need a customized strategy to be safe and successful.

Evaluate the recommendations' lucidity and comprehensiveness. Every step of the treatment plan, together with the reasoning behind it and the anticipated results, should be explained by a reliable physician. Along with explaining why they think their suggested strategy is the greatest fit for your needs, they should go over other possibilities. This degree of specificity shows their proficiency and dedication to your welfare.

Take into account how receptive the expert is to criticism and changes. Your treatment regimen should be adaptable so that it can be changed in response to your skin's needs. A cooperative approach guarantees the greatest outcomes and a satisfying experience, where the specialist cherishes your input and is open to making adjustments as needed.

DEVELOPING A LONG-TERM PARTNERSHIP IN SKINCARE

For continuous skin care goals and to preserve healthy skin, it's helpful to build a long-term connection with your skincare specialist. Frequent visits enable the specialist to track the development of your skin, modify treatments as necessary, and handle any emerging issues. This ongoing treatment aids in the management of long-term illnesses and the avoidance of possible problems.

A long-term partnership that works well depends on open communication. Notify your skincare specialist of any changes to your general health, lifestyle, or skin. This knowledge is essential for modifying your skincare routine and guaranteeing that treatments continue to work. A proactive approach that creates a solid, cooperative collaboration is one in which you feel at ease sharing your wants and concerns.

Both sides' commitment and consistency are crucial. Respect the treatment plans and follow-up appointments that your doctor prescribes, and in exchange, you should anticipate reliable, excellent care. Over time, developing trust results in improved outcomes and a more customized skincare experience, which eventually helps you reach and sustain your skin health objectives.

CHAPTER TWELVE

FAQS & FREQUENTLY ASKED QUESTIONS

TAKING CARE OF SKIN SENSITIVITY ISSUES

It's important to make sure your skincare routine is mild and customized for your skin type, particularly if you have sensitive skin. Determine the triggers and sensitivity points on your skin first. Fragrances, harsh chemicals, and specific substances like alcohol or sulfates are examples of common irritants. Choose products with dermatologist testing and hypoallergenic labels since their formulations reduce the likelihood of allergic responses. Before complete use, patch test new items on a tiny section of your skin to help determine potential sensitivities.

Create a regimen that contains relaxing components such as oatmeal, chamomile, or aloe vera, which are well-known for their calming effects. To gauge your skin's reaction to new products or treatments, introduce them gradually. If irritation develops, stop using the product and see a dermatologist. Last but not least, using SPF-containing creams and antioxidants to shield your skin from environmental stresses like pollution and UV rays can gradually lessen sensitivity.

BUDGETING AND MANAGING TREATMENT COSTS

Having good skincare doesn't have to be expensive. Prioritize basic items first, such as sunscreen, moisturizers, and cleansers. Seek for products that are multifunctional or that contain active components such as hyaluronic acid or retinol that have several advantages. A larger concentration of active chemicals can produce better results and eliminate the need for several products, so think twice before sacrificing quality for quantity.

Examine less expensive options like generic brands or homemade remedies made with organic components like avocado, yogurt, or honey.

Set aside money in your budget for routine skincare upkeep, as well as sporadic expert services like chemical peels or facials for more profound resurfacing. Utilize sample sizes, loyalty plans, and sales to trial new goods without having to make upfront full-sized purchases. You may get good results for less money by carefully selecting and prioritizing your skincare purchases.

SAFETY ADVICE FOR DO-IT-YOURSELF TREATMENTS

DIY skincare can be enjoyable and inexpensive, but safety must always come first to prevent negative responses. Make sure all components and recipes are safe for your skin type by doing extensive research on them. To stop allergies and contamination, sterilize containers and utensils. Before applying DIY remedies to your face or body, test the compatibility on a small patch of skin.

When following a recipe, don't make any substitutions unless a skincare expert recommends them. When using substances like essential oils, use caution as they can be highly concentrated and, if not diluted properly, cause skin irritation. For homemade goods, keep an eye on their expiration dates and throw away those that appear to be spoiling. When in doubt, seek advice from a dermatologist before beginning a do-it-yourself regimen, particularly for complicated conditions like hyperpigmentation or acne.

RECOGNIZING POSSIBLE ADVERSE EFFECTS

Making informed selections is facilitated by becoming knowledgeable about the possible adverse effects of skincare procedures. Retinoids, for example, frequently cause dryness, redness, and increased susceptibility to sunlight as adverse effects. Depending on the degree of the chemical peel and how well your skin tolerates it, temporary redness, peeling, or minor irritation may result from the procedure. Following a laser treatment, there may be brief edema, redness, or textural changes to the skin.

Before beginning treatments, always discuss potential side effects with a skincare expert. Carefully adhere to the post-treatment directions to reduce discomfort and maximize outcomes. Keep a watchful eye on your skin's response and let your dermatologist know right once if anything unexpected happens. Managing any side effects becomes an essential aspect of your skincare path toward healthier, more beautiful skin with the right planning and knowledge.

LONG-TERM ADVANTAGES AND UPKEEP

To achieve and sustain long-term skincare results, patience and consistency are essential. Create a regimen that includes cleansing, exfoliation, hydration, and UV protection based on the needs of your skin. Using skincare products with active compounds such as SPF, peptides, and antioxidants regularly helps preserve the suppleness and health of the skin.

Professional procedures like microdermabrasion, microneedling, and facials can enhance your everyday routine by addressing certain issues like fine lines or acne scars. Make appropriate adjustments to your skincare program as your skin changes with age and environmental conditions. Keep up with new developments in technology and products that could address your skin type and issues. With consistent effort and adaptation to your skin's changing requirements, you can experience long-lasting enhancements in the texture, tone, and general appearance of your skin.